Covid-19 and Vaccines Answers on Questions

Amanda Smith

Copyrights

© Copyright 2021 by *Amanda Smith.* All rights Reserved. No part of this publication or the information in it may be quoted from or reproduced in any form by means such as printing, scanning, photocopying or otherwise without prior written permission of the copyright holder.

Table of Contents:

Introduction _____ 5

What is COVID-19? _____ 7

Methods of infection _____ 9

How to protect yourself from infection? _____ 13

Vaccination against COVID-19 _____ 17

Moderna vaccine _____ 21

Pfizer and BioNTECH vaccine _____ 25

How long will immunity last? _____ 29

Conclusion _____ 33

Introduction

Today, one of the most actively discussed topics is COVID-19, that has changed the life of all people on the planet. There are many questions to which there are no answers. People are in fear, confusion, and complete disorientation of actions. Based on the research of the World Health Organization, it became known that COVID-19 becomes the cause of morbidity in all segments of the population, regardless of age or race. As a result of the massive morbidity, today we are forced to fight a rapidly developing epidemic. Unfortunately, medical scientists do not have complete data on the course of the disease, the symptoms of COVID-19, the mode of transmission, and prevention. Active development is underway to create an effective vaccine that will help fight the disease.

The main idea of the article is to inform the population with the necessary information about COVID-19, that refers to acute diseases, the causative agent of which

Introduction

is the SARS-CoV-2 coronavirus. In the book, I tried to give comprehensive information about the disease. Consequences and also indicate possible ways to prevent it.

You will also be able to find out all the details about vaccination against COVID-19 since the book pays special attention to this topic. Has all the data about the effectiveness of the vaccine been collected, all its characteristics have been considered, companies have been studied that are preparing to supply their developments to different countries of the world for mass vaccination of the population?

I will be glad if this article helps. Learn useful information about COVID-19. Reading the book, you will draw your conclusions and conclusions about the danger and severity of this virus, as well as learn the latest information on the development of a vaccine against COVID-19.

What is COVID-19?

So what is this COVID? After a long study, scientists call coronaviruses a virus that has been found in humans, as well as in some animals. It is quite common for the coronavirus to cause airway inflammation. But it was the SARS and MERS coronaviruses that caused very serious clinical cases that have a detrimental effect on the body. The SARS-CoV-2 virus has sufficient genetic material similarity to the SARS coronavirus.

The new coronavirus SARS-CoV-2 was caused by the well-known disease COVID-19. For the first time, the World Health Organization recorded information about this virus on December 31, 2019, after receiving information about the frequent cases of acute pneumonia caused by the virus in Wuhan, (China).

The symptoms of COVID-19 are quite nonspecific, and besides, they almost always differ due to the severity and characteristics of the human body. It can be com-

What is COVID-19?

pletely asymptomatic, it can also cause severe pneumonia, and in the worst case, COVID-19 can be fatal.

Methods of infection

The most common way of contracting a coronavirus infection is by airborne transmission, through direct contact with the carrier. When sneezing, coughing, or just talking, particles of the virus can get on the surface of the skin, eyes, nose, and mouth. Much less often, contaminated surfaces and surfaces with traces of the virus can be the cause of virus infection. According to the latest scientific research, COVID-19 can be stored indoors for up to 3 days at a comfortable temperature. Virus particles can be easily removed from surfaces by wet cleaning with disinfectants that can destroy the virus.

The average time for symptoms of COVID-19 to appear after contact with an infected person can vary from 5 to 6 days, but this period can also be from one to fourteen days. To reduce the spread of the coronavirus, individuals who have been in contact with infected individuals

Methods of infection

are urged to adhere to a self-isolation regime for two weeks.

Symptoms of COVID-19:

- dry cough;
- the feeling of weakness;
- increased body temperature;
- partial or complete loss of taste or smell;
- headache;
- sore throat;
- body aches;
- a feeling of nasal congestion;
- redness of the eyes;
- diarrhea;
- skin rash.

If you notice similar symptoms in yourself, we strongly recommend you do not neglect the health of yourself and your loved ones, and consult a doctor who will tell you how to act in this situation. Be sure to stay at home,

Methods of infection

do not expose other people to possible danger. Do not hesitate to seek medical help, because the earlier the disease is diagnosed, the less risks you will have.

By October 1, 2020, no special treatment regimen for COVID-19 was developed just as there was no known prevention method. Based on the data on October 16, 2020, in difficult situations, drugs such as corticosteroids were used to treat patients (October 16, 2020).

In 80% of cases, the disease is mild, there is no need to go to the hospital or take serious medications. Most people tolerate the disease easily, some have a mild illness similar to a cold. The risk group includes people with severe chronic diseases, those with asthma, diabetes, cancer, cardiovascular or autoimmune diseases, as well as elderly people. Their disease is very difficult usually, they need hospitalization, intensive therapy, and constant medical supervision. Light artificial ventilation devices and other devices are often used to support the work of vital organs.

How to protect yourself from infection?

To effectively reduce the infection of humanity with COVID-19, every person must know the rules of prevention and use the methods of protection that the Ministry of Health advises us. In total, there are several basic recommendations, all of which relate to hygiene. It is necessary to regularly wash your hands, rinse your nose, wear a protective mask in crowded places, and try to minimize being in crowds.

Here's how the World Health Organization has prepared precautions to prevent an increase in COVID-19 cases:

- You must wear a mask when you leave the house. For safety reasons, this recommendation should not be applied to children under 5 years of age. After all, a child cannot put on or take off the mask on his own, he can only make it worse, for example, touching it with dirty hands. Children

How to protect yourself from infection?

from 6 to 11 years old may not wear a mask if the area in which they live has not fallen into the epicenter of the spread of the virus. Also, children may not wear a mask due to the environment and school requirements. Teenagers (children from 12 years old) are required to wear a mask.

- It is necessary to be at a distance of half a meter from each other in a crowded place for the safety of you and those around you (this applies to queues, shopping, hospitals, etc.)

- Be sure to cover yourself when you sneeze. To do this, you can use a napkin or sneeze into the bend of your elbow.

- At the time of the epidemic, try to minimize staying in crowded places.

- You should ventilate the room.

How to protect yourself from infection?

- Be sure to wash your hands frequently and with soap.

- Use sanitizer for your hands.

In each region, additional rules and recommendations may apply, depending on the degree of infection of the population, climatic conditions, and others.

Vaccination against COVID-19

One might wonder why the COVID-19 vaccine needs to be used when you can just be careful to prevent getting the virus? The answer is very simple. People do not have developed immunity against the new strain that causes COVID-19, they can be infected anywhere and anyone, not an exception. and older people. Therefore, vaccination of the entire population and the acquisition of resistance to the virus will become a plus to the prevention and prevention of virus infection.

The main characteristic feature of COVID-19 is that it can penetrate a cell of human genetic material and reproduce there using human gene matter. Therefore, the RNA vaccine, which scientists all over the world are working on, must have the properties of recognizing the virus and prevent its particles from settling in the body.

The vaccine will work on the principle of forming antibodies capable of clearing out the virus and preventing it from hardening in the cells of the human body. Thus,

Vaccination against COVID-19

the coronavirus will be completely neutralized, and the person will be protected from disease.

"WHO" estimates that by the end of 2021 it will be possible to vaccinate only 20% of the world's population, so there is no need to put off masks, sanitizers, and gloves for now. We will keep our distance and quarantine measures for a long time.

Next, we will review the already created vaccines from various companies around the world.

Today, almost all developed countries strive to invent an effective vaccine against coronavirus faster than in other countries. Around the world, the development of the SARS-CoV-2 vaccine is at its peak. Large laboratories scattered around the globe trying to get the perfect vaccine in order. About 170 people are being voluntarily tested for the vaccine.

Vaccination against COVID-19

In the fall of 2020, the US company Moderna, the German corporation Pfizer, in partnership with Biontech, announced the creation of a working vaccine against coronavirus.

Moderna vaccine

The well-known company Moderna, headquartered in the United States, managed to create a vaccine that can protect humanity from COVID-19. During the creation of the vaccine, innovative techniques and the latest technologies were used, which allowed the creation of high-quality drugs in the largest possible amount in a short period.

The main feature and novelty of this technique is the use of messenger RNA. The whole point of this idea is to force the body to produce antibodies to the virus in the form of proteins similar to its own.

The test vaccination carried out showed that the mRNA-1273 vaccine from Moderna helps in 94.5% of cases, and in case of a severe course of the disease, it will help 100%. The vaccine can relieve symptoms and reduce the risk of death.

Moderna vaccine

This vaccine is used 2 times, 28 days should pass between the first and second injections. After applying the vaccine, a person acquires resistance to the virus for more than 3 months.

More than 30 thousand volunteers have experienced the effects of the vaccine. In this experiment, both the real vaccine and placebo were used for the purity of the results. As a result of the study, of the total number of volunteers, 95 people fell ill with Covid-19, 5 of whom were vaccinated with this vaccine. And it was in these 5 people that the disease cleared without complications.

One in ten subjects experienced temporary side effects such as redness of the skin at the injection site, headaches, and muscle aches.

To store the Moderna vaccine, extreme freezing is not needed, it will be enough only to maintain the temperature in the shipping container at least - 20 degrees. The vaccine is stored in a refrigerator, and subject to all temperature standards, it is suitable for use within 1 month after creation.

The vaccine will become publicly available after it has passed all the stages of research, testing and quality control in America.

It is worth remembering: for the effective effect of the vaccine on the body, and to prevent infection, it is necessary to inject two injections with an interval of 28 days.

Moderna says it will be able to produce approximately 500 million to billion doses of vaccines by the end of 2021.

Cost of vaccine

The approximate price of the Moderna vaccine will be around $ 25- $ 37.

Pfizer and BioNTECH vaccine

Pfizer and BioNTECH vaccine

The Pfizer / BioNTech vaccine is an innovative development from two impressive pharmaceutical corporations representing American manufacturers (Pfizer) and a German company (BioNTech). After qualitative research, the developers of the vaccine concluded that the effectiveness of the drug they created is 95%, immediately after applying two doses of the vaccine with a three-week interval.

The main weapon against coronavirus is the RNA vaccine, which performs its function thanks to a fragment of the virus genome. It is placed in a special shell, after vaccination, the genome enters the body and awakens the immune defense. Resistance to the disease is developed through the collision of the genome with the virus. 42,000 volunteers took part in Pfizer's Phase 3 Vaccine Study. 50% of the subjects received the actual vaccine, while others were injected with a placebo. The vaccine, from a joint partnership of a German and

Pfizer and BioNTECH vaccine

American company to BioNTech and Pfizer, has been officially recognized by the FDA as an effective and safe drug.

Also, special emphasis is made on the fact that based on 38 thousand successfully vaccinated subjects, it can be concluded that the drug is completely safe and ready to be used for mass protection against coronavirus. Also, it can be safely used in critical situations. Moreover, the FDA has assured that even after the first injection, the chance of contracting coronavirus is significantly reduced. These data were compiled based on long-term medical research and testing.

This drug has received the green light in the United Kingdom and Canada.

How does the vaccine work?

Pfizer provided a double injection technique with a 3-week break. Studies show that immunity will become resistant to the virus within a week after the second vaccination. Transportation became an acute problem

Pfizer and BioNTECH vaccine

in the distribution of the vaccine. This drug must be stored only at -70 degrees since the RNA and lipid vesicles included in it are rather unstable. But, fortunately, this problem was solved very quickly. For the successful transportation of the vaccine, it s suggested to use special coolers with GPS-tracking, f lled with dry ice. After the injection is completely defrosted, the bottle can be stored in the refrigerator for no more than 5 days. Already diluted and prepared, the bottle retains its properties for 6 hours and no more.

BioNTech and Pfize have already begun developing an improved vaccine that will not require such harsh storage conditions and will be resistant to higher temperatures.

How long will immunity last?

This is one of the most popular questions, to which no pharmaceutical company can give an exact answer. An indicator of how long your body will be resistant to the coronavirus will be an indicator for periodically repeating your vaccination. Only over time will we be able to find out what a person will need to resist the virus and how often he will need to repeat the injection. Will it be once every six months, a year, or for the whole life.

Based on recent studies, we can conclude that the body's resistance to the virus can last for a long time since most of the subjects and those who have had Covid-19 retain "immune memory" and antibodies to the strain.

Nevertheless, despite all the assurances of doctors and vaccine developers, the safety of the injection remains under big questions. This is especially true for children, the elderly, and pregnant women.

How long will immunity last?

Will the vaccine have a positive effect on children and older people?

Corporations declare that the effectiveness of vaccination does not depend on the age of the person, and even more so on his genetic or ethnic predisposition. Statistics show that approximately 94% of elderly people over the age of 60 have received a positive effect from the vaccine.

The subjects did not complain of ailments and side effects, only 3% of people experienced fatigue and headaches.

But what about children? Will children get adequate protection from the vaccine?

This question still has no clear answer. After all, initially, the age of the subjects was at least 18 years old, only then, 16-year-old teenagers began to take part in the research. They have already begun to test children over 12 years old. Thus, it is planned to systematically reduce the age limit during research

What will be the price of the future vaccine?

The company is in no hurry to disclose the final price of the drug. But, it was calculated that, on average, one vaccine would have to pay about $ 20. That is, the price of a full course of vaccination will not cost more than $ 40.

Conclusion

It can be stated that reducing the incidence and spread of Covid-19 is possible only by preventing the incidence. The number of cases will decrease significantly if all precautions are taken, adhering to quarantine, and gradual vaccination of the entire population. After the news about the creation of a vaccine, there was confidence that soon we would be able to completely eradicate Covid-19 and return to our usual way of life without fear for our health.

Unfortunately, there is still no 100% accurate information about the absolute effectiveness of the vaccine for all people. For example, the situation of children and people of the age remains in question. Plus, there is no exact certainty that the vaccine not only protects a person from the disease but also does not make him a carrier of the causative virus. There is no exact certainty how long the immunity will be resistant to the coronavirus after vaccination. It is suspected that the injec

Conclusion

tions will need to be repeated every year at best. It will take more than one year to provide the entire population with a vaccine. All of this shows that more detailed research, testing, and refinement are still required. Let's hope for the best and believe in the progressiveness of our medicine.

www.ingramcontent.com/pod-product-compliance
Lightning Source LLC
Chambersburg PA
CBHW031559210526
45464CB00003B/1341